Nature's Healers

A Comprehensive Guide to Herbal Medicine

Table of Contents

Chapter 1. Introduction

In this invigorating Special Report, "Nature's Healers: A Comprehensive Guide to Herbal Medicine," we delve into the lush green world of Mother Nature's pharmacy. Not only elevating your understanding of the abundant healing resources nature provides, it also stirs a newfound appreciation for the harmony existing between us and the world around us. From classic herbs to the less known gems of the botanical sphere, we cover both their medicinal virtues and safe application. Designed for everyone from novices to experts, the report delicately balances technical know-how with essential user-friendly information. With each page, we assure you, you'll feel empowered, energized, and more in tune with nature. Don't miss this golden opportunity to discover the healing powers that lie within humble leaves and roots – all it takes is this one Special Report to start your journey towards a healthier, herb-infused lifestyle!

Chapter 2. Herbal Medicine: A Brief Historical Overview

The path of herbal medicine is one that winds back across the ages, entwining itself through the annals of human history like the roots of a healing willow tree. From the cradle of civilization to the present day, plants have been both our allies and our saviors, providing nourishment and natural remedies. This chapter will lead you through the garden of time, detailing key periods in the historical development of herbalism, while planting seeds of appreciation for the magnitude of this ancient practice.

2.1. Ancient Beginnings

The roots of herbal medicine can be traced back to the dawn of human civilization. Early evidence from archaeological studies indicates human use of plants as medicine in the Paleolithic era, approximately 60,000 years ago. These early humans relied heavily on the surrounding flora for survival, not only for sustenance but also for curing ailments. It's probable that through trial and error, our ancestors learned to identify beneficial plants, knowledge which was then transferred down generations.

The Sumerians, one of the oldest civilizations, left us evidence of their knowledge of plants and their uses in the form of clay tablets dating back to 2600 B.C. These tablets listed hundreds of medicinal plants like myrtle, incense, and thyme—still in use today—showcasing their sophisticated understanding of flora.

2.2. Egyptian Eons

Ancient Egyptians hold a particularly influential place in the historical narrative of herbal medicine. Papyrus records from around

1500 B.C. exhibit an impressive list of approximately 700 plant medicines including garlic, juniper, cannabis, aloe, and poppy.

The Ebers Papyrus, one of the oldest and most important medical papyri of ancient Egypt, contained spells and prayers alongside herbal cures, revealing that the Egyptians understood the interconnectivity of physical and spiritual health. Some of the plants recommended in these ancient scripts remain popular today in homeopathic remedies, demonstrating the enduring prowess of herbal medicine.

2.3. Greek and Roman Eras

The Greeks followed suit, basing much of their medical approach on Egyptian methods. The renowned physician Hippocrates (460-377 BC), often referred to as the Father of Medicine, promoted herbal remedies, advocating for the body's innate capacity for self-healing. His philosophy, centered around diet and the health benefits of certain plants, became the foundation for western medicine.

The Romans too, fortified the traditions of herbal medicine, managing to expand and elaborate on them. Dioscorides, a Greek physician in the Roman army, documented over 600 plant-derived medicines in his five-volume encyclopedia, 'De Materia Medica'. This significant work served as the cornerstone for European herbal medicinal knowledge until the late middle ages.

2.4. Ayurveda and Traditional Chinese Medicine (TCM)

There would be an egregious omission if the ancient practices of Ayurveda from India, and Traditional Chinese Medicine (TCM) from China were not mentioned. Termed as 'wholistic', these practices understood the individual as an integral part of nature and emphasized the balance of mind, body and spirit. Both identified hundreds of botanicals for medicinal use.

TCM, with its roots dating back as far as 3500 B.C., incorporated various body practices, dietary therapy, acupuncture, and a vast range of plant medicines. Simultaneously, the Ayurvedic system, dating back to 1500 BC, integrated lifestyle modifications, yoga, and a complex herbal pharmacopia.

2.5. Middle Ages to Modern Day

Fast forwarding to Europe during the Middle Ages, while many misconceptions about herbs and health circulated, the wisdom of herbal medicine was kept alive by herb gardens in monasteries. In the age of Renaissance, the famous botanist, physician and astrologer Paracelsus, pledged his allegiance to nature, pronouncing that "The art of healing comes from nature, not from the physician."

Herbal medicine averted decline with the advent of modern pharmaceuticals but went through a period of reduction. Nonetheless, the World Wars triggered a resurgence, with many turning back to natural remedies amidst a scarcity of drugs.

Now, in the 21st century, as awakenings towards a more organic and sustainable lifestyle ensue, interest in herbal medicine is rapidly regenerating, reminding us of the value in these ancient, trusted practices.

2.6. Wrap Up

Every civilization, every culture, has its array of herbal tales interwoven with its history. The timeline of herbal medicine is rich with diverse uses and practices. It's a testament to the effort of countless generations who have contributed to the synthesis of knowledge that we draw upon today. As we fit into this timeline today, we contribute to the ongoing journey of herbal medicine, one that continues to expand our understanding of the remarkable gifts available to us from Mother Nature's pharmacy.

Chapter 3. Botanical Basics: Decoding the Plant Kingdom

To set the foundation for your exploration into herbal medicine, we'll peer into the vast, verdant expanse of the plant kingdom. This initial foray will help understand not only the types of plants, but also the components that make them potent choices for healing. We elucidate the systems of plant classification, delve into the internal anatomy of plants, and discuss the essential significance of key constituents like terpenoids, alkaloids, glycosides, and polyphenolic compounds.

3.1. Plant Classification: Taxonomy and Nomenclature

Plant classification is a congruous system designated to assign every plant to its specific group. These groupings, known as taxonomic ranks, include kingdom, division, class, order, family, genus, and species. The two most important ranks in terms of plant identification and utilization in herbal medicine are genus and species. For instance, in Camellia sinensis (the plant responsible for green and black tea), 'Camellia' refers to the genus while 'sinensis' denotes the species. This classification allows us to accurately communicate about the specific plant we're referring to, crucial for safe therapeutic use.

3.2. The Plant's Wardrobe: Root, Stem, Leaf, Flower, and Seed

Though plants come in a myriad of shapes and sizes, they all possess the same fundamental parts: root, stem, leaf, flower, and seed.

Roots anchor plants to the ground, absorb water and nutrients from the soil. Medicinally, roots like turmeric and ginseng are revered for their powerful health benefits. Stems, the plant's scaffolding, transport water, and nutrients, and produce new living tissue. Many stems, such as those of Aloe vera, harbor therapeutic goodies. Leaves execute photosynthesis, producing food for the plant. They're also the source of much medicinal magic – think aromatic peppermint or nourishing nettle. Flowers, the reproductive organs, create seeds which develop into new plants. Many flowers, like echinacea or hibiscus, are herbal medicine stars. Finally, seeds often contain concentrated amounts of potent plant compounds. Think flaxseeds or milk thistle seeds.

3.3. Discerning Plant Families: Similar But Not The Same

Plant families are groups of plants that have certain attributes in common. By identifying these families, we can ascertain therapeutic consistencies - and inconsistencies - among their members. Take the Apiaceae family (carrot family), a group with both highly beneficial and lethal members. The precious dandelion finds its relatives in this family, yet so does the deadly hemlock. Remember, every plant is uniquely individual, even within its group, just as every person is unique within their family.

3.4. Plant Anatomy: Cells and Tissues

Plants are composed of cells and tissues, distinctly different from our own but nonetheless, an essential part of the plant's form and function. Plant cells have specific organelles, such as chloroplasts for photosynthesis and large central vacuoles for storing water and ions. Plant tissues are divided into three types: dermal (external covering), vascular (for transport), and ground (for storage and support).

Various plant tissues can have distinctive therapeutic applications. For example, the bark of willow (a type of dermal tissue) has been used for pain relief, while the vascular tissues in dandelion have marked diuretic properties.

3.5. Phytochemicals: The Medicinal Molecules of Plants

Plants have evolved to produce an array of secondary metabolites known as phytochemicals. These compounds are not essential for the plant's survival, but they protect the plant from pests and diseases. In humans, these molecules can induce powerful, beneficial biological effects.

Some key groups of phytochemicals are:

- Terpenoids: These aromatic compounds give many plants their scent. They have diverse medicinal properties - anti-inflammatory (salicin in willow bark), antimicrobial (thymol in thyme), or anticancer (taxol from the Pacific yew tree).

- Alkaloids: These nitrogen-rich molecules are often seen in defense roles within plants. In humans, alkaloids have strong physiological effects. For example, morphine (from opium poppy) is a potent analgesic, while quinine (from Cinchona tree) has been used against malaria.

- Glycosides: In these compounds, one or more sugars are linked to a non-sugar molecule. They're known for their therapeutic effects, e.g., cardiac glycosides from Digitalis purpurea (foxglove) used in heart medications.

- Polyphenols: These are large groups of compounds with varying structures, known primarily for antioxidant activity. They're abundant in tea, wine, and many fruits and veggies.

With this preliminary understanding of the botanical basics, you're well-equipped to navigate your journey into the fascinating world of herbal medicine. The potent healing power of a plant is not only in its leaf, stem, root, flower, or seed, but intricately tied to its unique taxonomy, anatomy, and the complex medley of phytochemicals each plant possesses.

Chapter 4. Top 20 Essential Herbs: Profiles and Uses

As we venture into the vivid green landscape of herbal medicine, we unveil the profound wisdom encapsulated in plants, observing the unique characteristics and healing abilities of each herb. Our journey unfolds with the exploration of the top 20 essential herbs that every herbal medicine devotee must know.

4.1. 1. Basil

Basil (**Ocimum basilicum**) is a classic kitchen herb that transcends its culinary use. Its leaf contains potent essential oils, such as eugenol, known for its anti-inflammatory and antibacterial properties. It proves beneficial in treating digestion issues, respiratory problems, and it may also check mental exhaustion and mild depression.

4.2. 2. Chamomile

Chamomile, available in two species— Roman (**Chamaemelum nobile**) and German (**Matricaria recutita**)— is revered for its calming effects. Often infused into teas, the flowers combat insomnia, aid in digestive wellness, soothe skin irritations, and boost the immune system.

4.3. 3. Echinacea

Echinacea (**Echinacea** spp.) root and flowering tops are popular for their potential to boost immunity. Traditional use supports their ability to shorten the duration of colds and treat upper respiratory infections.

4.4. 4. Garlic

Garlic (**Allium sativum**) is a potent antimicrobial agent. It's useful in battling infections, lowering blood pressure, reducing cholesterol levels, and possibly improving cardiovascular health.

4.5. 5. Ginger

Ginger (**Zingiber officinale**) roots offer relief from nausea, motion sickness, and digestion-related ailments. Its anti-inflammatory properties also provide relief from pain and swelling.

4.6. 6. Ginkgo

Ginkgo (**Ginkgo biloba**) leaf is traditionally used to treat memory disorders, improve circulation, reduce age-related macular degeneration, and relieve PMS symptoms.

4.7. 7. Ginseng

Ginseng root, available in various species like Asian (**Panax ginseng**) and American (**Panax quinquefolius**), is hailed for enhancing stamina, reducing fatigue, managing stress, and possibly taming diabetes.

4.8. 8. Lavender

The fragrant flowers of Lavender (**Lavandula** spp.) possess calming properties and contribute to healing burns, cuts, and other skin issues besides promoting sound sleep.

4.9. 9. Lemon Balm

Lemon balm (**Melissa officinalis**) leaves are beneficial for soothing the nerves, promoting sleep, treating wounds, and enhancing memory and alertness.

4.10. 10. Marjoram

Marjoram (**Origanum majorana**) leaf can ease digestive issues, reduce inflammation, and help in managing hormones and menstrual problems.

4.11. 11. Milk Thistle

Milk Thistle (**Silybum marianum**) seeds are commonly used for liver detox, improving liver function and treating liver disorders.

4.12. 12. Nettle

Stinging Nettle (**Urtica dioica**) leaf is a treasure trove of nutrition and helps in chronic inflammation, allergies, and arthritis.

4.13. 13. Peppermint.

The leaves of Peppermint (**Mentha piperita**) can relieve a variety of digestive issues like IBS and nausea. This plant also aids in respiration issues and can alleviate headache pain.

4.14. 14. Rosemary.

Rosemary (**Rosmarinus officinalis**) leaf is an antioxidant power center. It is used for digestion problems, improving memory, and relieving muscle pain and spasm.

4.15. 15. Sage

Sage (**Salvia officinalis**) leaf handles digestion problems, provides relief from menstrual cramps, reduces sweating, and improves cognitive function.

4.16. 16. Thyme

Thyme (**Thymus vulgaris**) leaf is utilized as an antibacterial and antifungal agent. It's also useful in respiratory health, boosting immunity, and promoting good digestion.

4.17. 17. Turmeric

The root of Turmeric (**Curcuma longa**) boasts potent anti-inflammatory effects. It's also used for improving digestion, enhancing liver function, and possibly providing relief from arthritic pain.

4.18. 18. Valerian

Valerian (**Valeriana officinalis**) root eases sleeping disorders, anxiety, and menstrual cramps.

4.19. 19. Witch Hazel

Witch Hazel (**Hamamelis virginiana**) bark and leaf are excellent in reducing skin inflammation and treating hemorrhoids, minor burns, and skin irritation.

4.20. 20. Yarrow

Yarrow (**Achillea millefolium**) flowering tops exhibit anti-inflammatory, analgesic, and anti-bleeding effects. It treats wounds, burns, rashes, and aids in digestive health.

As we delve deeper into the mystic world of nature, it's important to remember that whilst herbs are powerful healers, they should always be used responsibly. Consultation with a health care professional before starting any new herbal regimen is a necessity, especially for pregnant, nursing women, children, and those with pre-existing medical conditions. This ensures that you reap the maximum benefit from Mother Nature's wisdom without any adverse effects.

A profound exploration of nature's botanical treasures invites you, stirring a newfound appreciation for the harmony that exists between us and the world around us. Grasping the lore of these top 20 essential herbs, you are now more equipped to embark on a journey towards a healthier, herb-infused lifestyle.

Chapter 5. Preparing Herbal Remedies: Infusions, Decoctions, and Tinctures

Unearthing the age-old wisdom of herbal remedies, we explore three primary processes through which the potency of herbs can be extracted for use - Infusions, Decoctions, and Tinctures. Mastering these basic herbal preparation methods will empower you to harness the healing powers of plants for your wellness needs.

5.1. The Art of Infusions

An infusion is a potent water-based method used to extract the medicinal properties of herbs. Being gentle, it is perfect for delicate parts of the plant such as leaves, flowers, and aromatic herb parts.

To prepare an infusion, gather fresh or dried herbs, choosing organically grown varieties whenever possible. Infuse one teaspoon of dried or one tablespoon of fresh herbs in one cup of boiling water. Allow the mixture to steep for 10 to 20 minutes, strain, and enjoy. Use a ceramic, glass, or stainless teapot to prevent an undesired chemical reaction. Cover while steeping to preserve the volatile oils. Sip the infusion while it is warm, up to three times a day. Note that infusions have a short shelf life and should ideally be consumed within 24 hours.

For a cold infusion, steep herbs in cold water for a longer period, usually several hours or overnight. This method is suitable for herbs that contain active compounds that can be destroyed by heat.

5.2. From Brew to Decoctions

Decoctions are for the heavier plant materials such as roots, bark, heavy seeds, and berries. These parts usually require additional heat to more thoroughly break down plant material and release medicinal qualities.

For preparing a decoction, take one tablespoon of dried herbs or two tablespoons of fresh herbs per cup of water. Place the herbs in a pot, add cold water, and bring to a boil slowly. Let it simmer for 15 to 30 minutes, depending on the hardiness of the plant material. Strain the residue, ensuring no herb parts remain. Decoctions, like infusions, should be consumed warm and within a day to assure potency.

5.3. Elixir of Life: Tinctures

The endurance runner of herbal remedies, tinctures involve steeping herbs in alcohol to create a long-lasting and potent remedy. Tinctures ensure that even the most stubborn beneficial compounds are extracted, and the longer shelf life (up to several years) allows for preservation and convenience.

First, fill a jar 1/3 to 1/2 full with dried herbs. You may need to adjust the quantity depending on the fluffiness or denseness of the herb. Pour alcohol over the herbs, completely covering them by at least two inches. Use an 80 to 100 proof vodka or brandy for optimal results.

Next, cover the jar and store in a cool, dark place for at least six weeks. Shake occasionally during this period. After six weeks, strain the mixture through a fine mesh strainer or cheesecloth, ensuring that all plant material has been removed. Store the tincture in an amber glass bottle out of direct sunlight.

Many herbalists prefer to use a dropper for administering tinctures, as this allows for flexible and accurate dosing. The generally recommended dose for tinctures is 1-2 ml, three times a day, diluted in a small amount of water.

5.4. Exploring Variety: Mixed-Methods

There's also room for exploration and variation in preparing herbal remedies. Consider cold macerations for sensitive plants, infused oils for topical applications, or herbal honey for sweet and soothing care. The world of herbal remedies is a diverse one, with no 'one-size-fits-all.' The key is to fully understand the nature of herbs and the best method to unlock their medicinal powers.

In this chapter, we understood the crucial processes of preparing herbal medicine - Infusion, decoction, and tincture. They serve as the backbone of any herbal remedy repertoire and a stepping stone to a therapeutic, symbiotic relationship with the plant kingdom. As we indulge in these rituals of preparation, let us remember to honor the wisdom of the herbs and the energy they carry, taking time to understand their properties, harvesting responsibly, and treating each plant with the respect it deserves. Happy brewing!

Chapter 6. Safety and Precautions: Interactions and Contraindications

Before diving headfirst into the exciting world of herbal medicine, it's essential to fully understand how this alternative therapy may interact with other aspects of your overall health regime, its contraindications and potential risk factors involved. So, let's embark on this crucial part of your herbal journey.

6.1. Understanding Herbal Interactions

An interaction, in the context of herbal medicine, refers to the effect a herb might have when used alongside other medications. Herbal interactions might either boost or diminish the effect of your conventional medicines, impacting its therapeutic outcome.

Take, for example, St. John's wort, a herb famous for its mood-lifting properties. It can interact with a myriad of prescription drugs including antidepressants, contraceptives, and anticoagulants, often resulting in decreased efficacy of these substances.

Now, it's not always the case that an interaction is detrimental. Some carefully executed pairings can enhance therapeutic benefits. In fact, some herbs when taken with certain vitamins, minerals, or other supplements can elevate their absorption by the body. An instance of such a beneficial interaction is the pairing of black pepper with turmeric. The piperine in black pepper enhances the absorption of curcumin, the active compound in turmeric, up to 2000%.

The interactions of herbal medicine are largely dependent on the individual herbs involved, the dosage, the manner of administration and the person receiving the treatment. That's why, in pursuing herbal treatments it's important to be openly communicative with your healthcare provider so they can monitor any potential interactions and adjust your treatment accordingly.

6.2. Contraindications and Adverse Effects

While herbs are natural, they are not necessarily benign. Certain conditions or factors may render a person unsuitable for certain herbal treatments. This idea gives rise to the theory of contraindications in herbal medicine.

For instance, pregnant and breastfeeding women are usually advised to steer clear of several herbs like mugwort, pennyroyal, and tansy due to their potential to induce miscarriage or negatively impact milk supply. Certain individuals might also have allergies to specific herbs which could result in adverse skin reactions, gastrointestinal issues, and respiratory complications.

Moreover, some herbs can cause adverse effects. For instance, although Milk Thistle is heralded for its liver-protective properties, it may cause nausea, bloating, and diarrhea in some individuals. In addition, prolonged use of Cascara sagrada, a well-known herbal laxative, may lead to electrolyte and fluid imbalances in your body.

Potential adverse effects should be viewed as reminders to approach herbal medicine with informed caution rather than to deter you from using them.

6.3. Safe and Responsible Use of Herbal Medicine

Having touched on the important notions of interactions and contraindications, let's now consider some practical guidance for a safe and responsible journey into herbal healing.

Always begin by seeking advice from trained herbalists or naturopaths. Get thorough information about appropriate dosages, preparation methods, and potential side effects. Never exceed suggested dosages. Like any medicine, an overdose of herbal treatment can be harmful.

It's also beneficial to familiarize oneself with reliable holistic health information sources and maintain a dialogue with your healthcare provider about your herbal supplements. This step ensures you correctly understand the benefits and risks associated with your herbal treatment.

When purchasing herb-related products, pay attention to labels. Look for products having seals of approval from recognized bodies that verify the product quality, such as the U.S. Pharmacopeia, NSF International, or ConsumerLab.

As we journey deeper into this herbal wonderland, the key is to be mindful and aware. Use this knowledge as your compass navigating you through the lush green landscape of herbal medicine, savoring its sweet fruits while sidestepping potential pitfalls along the way. With prudence and informed respect, we can surely beckon the healing touch of nature into our lives.

Chapter 7. Herbs for Common Ailments: From Colds to Anxiety

Before delving into the wide array of herbs that nature generously endows upon us for our wellness, it is essential to instill a strong preventive mindset. While herbs are excellent at treating many common ailments, the best way to live a healthy life is through healthy living habits: a balanced diet, moderate exercise, good sleep, and a positive mental attitude.

That being said, even the healthiest of individuals encounter mild illnesses or experience stress-related issues. Here, herbal remedies come in, offering a gentle yet effective solution that harmonizes with our body's intrinsic healing mechanisms.

Let's explore some herbs that mitigate the impact of typical health concerns from colds to anxiety, including their therapeutic properties, preparation methods, and application guidelines.

7.1. Herbs for the Common Cold

The common cold, as ubiquitous as it may seem, is an ailment we have all encountered. Plagued by stuffy noses, coughs, and general malaise, our day can get arduous. However, the plant kingdom offers effective solutions.

1. **Echinacea**: This purple flower has earned its reputation as a cold-fighting powerhouse due to its immune-boosting effects. Echinacea tea or tincture can be taken at the first sign of a cold to expedite recovery.

2. **Elderberry**: Elderberries, when consumed in the form of a syrup, can reduce cold duration and severity. Packed with antioxidants,

they bolster the immune system and combat the cold virus.

3. **Ginger**: A cup of ginger tea infused with honey and lemon can break down the congestion and soothe a sore throat.

7.2. Herbs for Digestive Disorders

Digestive issues like indigestion, bloating, or constipation can play havoc with our comfort and well-being. Luckily, we have time-honored herbal remedies at our disposal.

1. **Peppermint**: Known for its refreshing flavor, peppermint soothes stomach muscles, reducing bloating and abdominal pain. A warm cup of peppermint tea post-meal can work wonders for digestion.

2. **Chamomile**: Much more than a calming tea, chamomile can alleviate digestive discomfort by reducing inflammation and acidity.

3. **Fennel**: Fennel seeds, brewed as a tea or chewed directly, work as an excellent digestive aid, easing bloating and gas.

7.3. Herbs for Anxiety and Stress

In the face of constant stressors from our fast-paced lifestyle, mental well-being is paramount. Here, again, Mother Nature lends a hand.

1. **Ashwagandha**: An esteemed herb of Ayurveda, ashwagandha is an adaptogenic herb that helps the body manage stress better.

2. **Lavender**: The mere scent of lavender can reduce anxiety and promote sleep. Lavender sachets, essential oil, or an infusion in tea can integrate this calming herb into your routine.

3. **Lemon Balm**: This fragrant herb uplifts mood, reduces anxiety, and promotes a sense of calm. You can enjoy its benefits in the form of tea or as an essential oil.

Remember, herbs, while wonderfully beneficial, are not a substitute for medical treatment. Always consult with a healthcare provider before starting any herbal regimen. Also, remember to source organic, high-quality herbs to truly reap the advantages they can bestow upon us.

As this exploration into the world of herbal remedies concludes, it's essential to understand that the journey does not. With knowledge as your guide and nature as your ally, the path to a healthier you is but a step away. Seek the knowledge, respect the plant kingdom, and relish the journey!

Chapter 8. Kitchen Pharmacy: Cooking with Healing Herbs

Of all the rooms in our homes, the kitchen holds the most potential to strengthen our wellbeing through the food we eat. In this bustling culinary workroom, healthful herbs can be put to use as deliciously therapeutic additions, delivering benefits far beyond mere flavor enhancement. Let us explore some kitchen staples and their remarkable healing properties.

8.1. Understanding the Importance of Herbal Culinary Arts

The art of cooking with herbs has roots in most culinary traditions worldwide. Whether it's soothing cilantro in Mexican cuisine, antioxidant-rich basil in Italian food, or healing garlic embraced by many food cultures, each herb carries its specific health properties into our diets, so unobtrusively. They are full of phytochemicals that may help prevent and combat various ailments. Far from alternative medicine, this is a lifestyle approach to naturally promote good health.

8.2. A Comprehensive List of Healing Herbs

Before diving into how we can use these verdant healers in our cuisine, let's familiarize ourselves with some common culinary herbs and their benefits.

1. **Basil:** Aids digestion, fights free-radical activity, and exhibits anti-inflammatory properties.

2. **Parsley:** Rich in Vitamin K, Vitamin C, and flavonoids, parsley has potent antioxidant and anti-inflammatory properties.

3. **Rosemary:** Known to enhance memory and concentration, it also has anti-inflammatory, antibacterial, and digestion-healing properties.

4. **Thyme:** A strong antiseptic, thyme can treat ailments like upset stomach, arthritis, and sore throat.

5. **Oregano:** Antioxidant-rich, oregano supports immune health and can fight bacteria.

This list is in no way exhaustive, as there's a world of medicinal herbs out there, waiting to be explored.

8.3. Infusing Your Everyday Meals

The key to incorporating healing herbs into your diet is to weave them seamlessly into your everyday meals. Here's how.

Salads: Tossing handfuls of fresh herbs like basil, parsley, and mint into salads isn't just refreshing; it's health-promoting too.

Smoothies: Putting herbs like mint or parsley in your smoothies delivers a flavor kick and a nutrient boost.

Herb-Infused Oils: Infuse your cooking oils with herbs like rosemary or thyme by heating them lightly together. Store and use in your cooking for an extra depth of flavor and health.

Rubs and Marinades: Mix finely chopped herbs with a little olive oil for a healing marinade or rub for meats or vegetables.

Herbal Teas: Sip on mint or chamomile tea for a gentle, calming effect or brew thyme tea to fight cold symptoms.

8.4. Proper Storage and Preservation of Herbs

To ensure maximum flavor and medicinal value, store herbs properly. Most herbs are best stored in the crisper drawer of your refrigerator, wrapped in a slightly damp paper towel inside a resealable bag.

Alternatively, you can freeze herbs. Chop them finely, place in an ice cube tray with a little water, and retrieve a cube when required. However, note that frozen herbs might lose some of their firm texture, making them better in cooked dishes than raw ones.

Herbs can also be dried but keep in mind that some herbs lose their flavor and medicinal effectiveness when dried. To dry herbs, hang them upside down in a cool, dry place until completely dry, then store in airtight containers away from light.

8.5. Moving Forward with Herbal Healing

It's vital to remember that while herbs can contribute significantly to our health, they should accompany a balanced diet and a healthy lifestyle. Also, consult a healthcare professional before using herbs therapeutically, especially if pregnant, nursing, or dealing with specific health conditions.

Begin with integrating a variety of these herbs into your meals. Try new recipes, experiment with different blends, and discover the potent combinations that appeal to your palate. With practice and creativity, your kitchen can truly transform into your personal pharmacy, wrapping wellness into every bite you take.

Remember, nature's healing power isn't locked away in rare, exotic plants alone. It's right there on your kitchen shelf, among the unassuming sprigs of parsley, in the fragrant leaves of basil, within the gnarled clove of garlic, and within every herb-infused meal you cook. Go forth – cook, eat, heal!

Chapter 9. Cultivating Your Herbal Garden: A Step-by-step Guide

Creating your own herbal garden can be a rewarding experience that not only brings the beauty of nature closer to home but also provides a convenient repository of healing plants just within your reach. Here, we explore the steps necessary to establish and flourish your very own herbal garden, from the selection of sites and herbs, to maintaining the plant's health and eventually using them for their therapeutic properties.

9.1. Choosing the Right Site

Before delving into the gardening aspect, it is vital to understand that the location of your herbal garden plays a crucial role in the success of your endeavor. Some aspects to consider are the hours of sunlight exposure, soil type, and accessibility. As a rule, most herbs prefer full sun (about 6-8 hours per day), well-drained soil that is rich in organic matter, and a location that's close to your kitchen or your area of use.

9.2. Selecting Your Herbs

The choice of herbs is dependent on your specific needs, both culinary and medicinal. Select herbs that are relevant to your health needs and ones that you would delight in growing. Some commonly cultivated medicinal herbs include Echinacea for boosting the immune system, chamomile for its calming effects, and peppermint for digestion and relaxing the mind.

9.3. Starting from Seeds or Plants

You have two main choices when starting your herbal garden: starting from seeds or buying plants. Starting from seeds may require additional time and attention. However, the greater diversity of plants is available in seed form. On the other hand, buying plants can give you a jump start, especially in short-growing season climates.

9.4. Planting Your Herbs

Whether you're working with seed or transplants, the planting process remains relatively the same. Dig a hole larger than the root ball of the plant, place the plant or seed in the hole, cover, and firm down gently. Water immediately to minimize transplant shock. Seeds will need to be started in small pots or seed starter trays before transplanting outside.

9.5. Caring for Your Herbal Garden

Herbal plants, like any other plants, require care and maintenance to induce optimal growth. Regular watering is crucial, but avoid overwatering as it could lead to root rot. Pruning helps to regulate the plant's growth, assures healthy circulation, and encourages new growth. Additionally, regular harvests, particularly for annuals, help herbs to stay productive.

9.6. Dealing with Pests and Diseases

Deterring pests and disease naturally maintains harmony in your garden. Certain plants act as repellants for specific pests, use this companion planting principle to protect your plants. Regular inspection of your plants will keep you proactive against potential pest infestations and diseases.

9.7. Harvesting Your Herbs

To ensure that your herbs maintain their medicinal properties, harvest them at the right time. Generally, herbs should be harvested before the plant starts to bloom, as at this stage, it contains a maximum concentration of essential oils. Use sharp pruners or scissors and avoid bruising the plant tissues.

9.8. Drying and Storing Herbs

After harvesting, drying is the most common way of preserving herbs. Air drying is the simplest method - just make sure to do it in a well-ventilated area away from direct sunlight. For storing, use air-tight containers, clearly label them with the name of the herb and the date of the harvest.

9.9. Using Your Herbs

Lastly, comes the reward of your hard labor. Whether you're using these herbs in cooking or brewing them into tea, make sure to research their usage beforehand. Some herbs offer amazing benefits when used fresh and others when brewed or even made into tinctures or oils.

Venturing into this journey of establishing your own herbal garden is not only an exciting personal project, but it also signifies a step towards a more holistic and health-driven lifestyle. As you cultivate these plants, you're also cultivating well-being and a deep sense of harmony with nature. It certainly invigorates the old saying, "Your food be your medicine and your medicine be your food."

Chapter 10. Herbal Medicine Around the World: Practices and Traditions

The breadth of herbal medicine practices is as varied and diverse as the cultures it hails from. Often passed down through generations, these methods of treatment weave tightly into local customs and traditions, reflecting the unique personality of each region's flora and fauna.

10.1. Asia

In Asia, herbal medicine takes on a mystic character. Rooted in centuries-old philosophies, these practices intertwine with spirituality and mystique, making for a unique healing endeavor.

10.1.1. Chinese Traditional Medicine

Chinese Traditional Medicine (CTM) is perhaps the most well-known Eastern practice, dating back to the very cradle of Chinese civilization. The fundamental Doctrine of Signatures posits that herbs resembling various parts of the body can be used to heal ailments specific to those body parts.

CTM utilizes a wide range of herbs, often in combination, to restore the body's essential balance. Ginseng is a quintessential representation, lauded for its rejuvenating properties. Similarly, astragalus, angelica, and licorice root are fundamental to many herbal concoctions used in CTM.

10.1.2. Ayurveda

An ancient practice from India, Ayurveda is less a method of treatment and more a philosophy of life. It posits that all things in the universe, including the human body, are made up of the five elements of space, air, fire, water, and earth. Balancing these elements through diet, lifestyle, meditation, and herbal remedies is central to Ayurvedic healing.

Noteworthy herbs in Ayurvedic medicine include turmeric, used for its anti-inflammatory properties; ashwagandha, a powerful adaptogen reducing stress and bolstering the immune system; Brahmi, a brain tonic; and Amla, a potent source of Vitamin C.

10.2. The Americas

Across the Atlantic, North and South America offer a distinct yet equally profound take on herbal treatments, steeped in Indigenous traditions.

10.2.1. Native American Medicine

Native American tribes utilized local plants for a vast range of purposes. They used white willow bark as a pain reliever, echinacea to boost immunity, and sage for purification. Many of these practices continue to be important within Native communities.

10.2.2. South American Traditions

South America, particularly the Amazon rainforest, boasts a myriad of active plants. For example, Cat's Claw has anti-inflammatory and antioxidant properties while Pau d'Arco treats infections and fevers. Perhaps most famous is ayahuasca, a powerful hallucinogenic brew with deep spiritual significance, used under the careful supervision of shamans.

10.3. Africa

In Africa, herbal medicine is a vital component of healthcare due to the continent's richness in medicinal plants and the lingering inaccessibility of modern medicine in some areas.

Ubulawu is a collection of cleansing and dream-inducing plants prevalent in Southern Africa, often used to communicate with ancestors. Meanwhile, in West Africa, the Voacanga Africana tree is widely recognized for its pain relief and stimulant properties.

10.4. Europe

European herbal tradition is rooted in two main veins: the classical Greek tradition, which prevailed until the Middle Ages, followed by a more scientific approach that emerged during the Renaissance.

10.4.1. Greek Tradition

The Greek physician Hippocrates valued a holistic approach, using herbs such as mint and marjoram for digestion, as well as willow bark for pain relief. Later, Galen introduced the concept of 'Galenical pharmacy', referring to the preparation of medicines from plants.

10.4.2. Modern European Herbalism

Today, herbalism in Europe is more regulated, with a major focus on scientific validation. St. John's Wort is used widely for treating mild to moderate depression, while Valerian is popular as a mild sedative.

Herbal medicine, while differing greatly across cultural lines, harbors a common thread - reliance on the bounty of nature for healing. Behind the cataloging of beneficial plants lies centuries of empirical knowledge, each tradition illuminating a different facet of the connection between humankind and nature.

Chapter 11. Future Trends: The Role of Herbal Medicine in Modern Healthcare

In the vibrant and bustling field of contemporary healthcare, one may find it astounding that herbal medicine, a form of therapy so deeply rooted in our planet's rich history, continues to play a pivotal role. However, the truth is that in an era characterized by groundbreaking technological and scientific advancements, herbal medicine continues not just to persist but to thrive and evolve.

Let's embark on a journey that investigates this unprecedented trend, trekking across the growing role of herbal medicine in today's healthcare, its multifarious applications, the intriguing mixture of traditional practices and modern science and, of course, an exploration of what the future might hold for this ancient art.

11.1. The Rising Popularity of Herbal Medicine

In the last few decades, the world has witnessed a renewed interest in herbal medicine. This revival is partly attributed to a growing disenchantment with mainstream allopathy and the damaging side-effects associated with some synthetic drugs. More and more people are turning towards nature for answers to their health woes, and researchers worldwide are increasingly noticing and investigating these phenomena.

According to a World Health Organization (WHO) report, around 80% of the world's population, especially those living in developing countries, rely on herbal medicine for their primary healthcare. Even in developed nations such as the US and Germany, nearly half of the population have used some form of complementary or alternative medicine, and herbal medicine forms a considerable part of this fraction.

11.2. A Fusion of Tradition and Modern Medicine

Modern medicine is beginning to realize the potential value rooted in traditional treatments. As such, an growing number of scientific studies are being conducted to validate the efficacy of these remedies, amalgamating two seemingly contradictory worlds - traditional knowledge and scientific methodologies.

Evidence-based herbal medicine is becoming the norm, with rigorous testing and analysis confirming the medicinal properties of plants previously esteemed solely by traditional healers. This shift has started to bridge the gap between herbalists and mainstream health professionals, leading to more integrated and holistic treatment approaches.

11.3. Applications in Modern Healthcare

A vast array of medicinal plants are finding their niche within modern healthcare. Below are some notable examples:

- **Turmeric (Curcuma longa)**: This golden spice, cherished in Indian Ayurvedic medicine, has been authenticated by modern science for its potent anti-inflammatory properties. It now finds mention in standard Western medical texts for its use in managing arthritic conditions.

- **St. John's Wort (Hypericum perforatum)**: A common herb used traditionally in the treatment of mild to moderate depression, St.

John's wort has been validated by several high-quality clinical trials that have shown efficacy comparable to standard antidepressants.

- **Ginkgo (Ginkgo biloba)**: The leaves of the ancient Ginkgo tree have stood the test of time, emerging as a promising therapeutic tool for dementia and memory impairments in numerous scientific studies.

- **Garlic (Allium sativum)**: From being added for flavor in cooking to serving as medicine, Garlic is appreciated for its applications in cardiovascular health, thanks to its ability to lower blood cholesterol levels and blood pressure.

11.4. The Role of Technology

Technological advancements have been instrumental in pushing forward the frontiers of herbal medicine. Methods such as phytochemical screening, genomics, proteomics, and metabolomics are now used to identify and quantify the active ingredients of medicinal plants. These processes have paved the way for the development of standardized herbal extracts that provide consistent and reproducible health benefits.

Moreover, the use of blockchain technology can help enhance quality control in the herbal medicine supply chain. This offers greater transparency in sourcing herbs and can aid in reducing the adulteration issue often plaguing the industry.

11.5. The Future of Herbal Medicine

Looking into the future, it is expected that herbal medicine will accumulate an even more significant role in healthcare. With an increasing body of scientific validation and technological solutions that ensure quality and efficacy, herbal medicine is well-positioned to become a critical element of personal health management strategies.

Furthermore, the integration of herbal medicine into mainstream healthcare practice can lead to more personalized, patient-centric care. Genetic profiling could give rise to personalized herbal treatments, based on an individual's unique genetic makeup.

As we venture deeper into the millennium, the growing trend of 'green prescriptions', where healthcare providers recommend nature-based activities and herbs for health promotion, is uplifting. It not only underpins the recognition of the immense therapeutic potential of the green world but also highlights a trend towards a more environmentally conscious and sustainable approach to health.

In conclusion, it is clear that the ancient craft of herbal medicine is finding its rightful place in the modern health domain. While the journey is still very much in its infancy, each step taken towards integrating nature's wisdom into contemporary medicine gives patients a further holistic, effective, and personalized health care strategy. Again, as this happens, it hails a more sustainable approach not just for humanity's health, but for the planet's health too.